RHEUMATOID ARTHRITIS (RA) COOKBOOK

Complete Dietary Suggestions For Rheumatoid Arthritis

Dr. ATHENA ABELL

Table of Contents

CHAPTER ONE

Introduction

Rheumatoid Arthritis (RA) is a persistent autoimmune disorder that impacts a substantial global population, manifesting as joint pain, inflammation, and rigidity.

Although medical interventions are of paramount importance in the management of the condition, recent studies have brought attention to the substantial influence that dietary decisions have on the progression and manifestation of symptoms associated with rheumatoid arthritis.

Anti-inflammatory diets have emerged as particularly promising adjunct therapies, providing individuals with rheumatoid arthritis with a proactive approach to supplement conventional treatments.

The present article delves into the correlation between Rheumatoid Arthritis, inflammation, and the critical significance of an anti-inflammatory diet, concentrating particularly on the integration of fruits and vegetables.

Inflammation and Rheumatoid Arthritis: A Comprehension

Rheumatoid Arthritis is distinguished by an erroneous assault by the immune system on the synovium, which comprises the lining of the membranes encircling the joints. This results in inflammation, which can affect other bodily systems and organs in addition to causing joint injury. Joint inflammation is a chronic condition that is implicated in the development of joint discomfort, edema, and the gradual deterioration of joint tissues.

Fundamentally, inflammation is the physiological reaction of the body to an infection or injury. In autoimmune conditions, such as rheumatoid arthritis, the inflammatory response becomes persistent and targets the tissues of the body. In addition to aggravating the symptoms of rheumatoid arthritis, this chronic inflammation may also result in irreversible joint injury.

The Value Of Consuming An Anti-Inflammatory Diet

By reducing inflammation in the body, an anti-inflammatory diet offers a holistic approach to the management of conditions such as rheumatoid arthritis. The principal objective is to include in one's diet foods that possess anti-inflammatory properties while avoiding those that could potentially exacerbate inflammation.

It has been suggested by a multitude of studies that diet significantly influences the regulation of inflammation. It has been discovered that foods abundant in phytonutrients, omega-3 fatty acids, and antioxidants possess anti-inflammatory properties. A diet abundant in refined carbohydrates, saturated fats, and processed foods, on the other hand, may contribute to inflammation.

Adopting an anti-inflammatory diet may potentially reduce the frequency and severity of flare-ups, improve joint function, and enhance overall well-being in individuals with rheumatoid arthritis (RA), in addition to supplementing medical treatments. Although diet cannot resolve rheumatoid arthritis on its own, it can have a substantial effect on the inflammatory processes that are linked to the condition.

CHAPTER TWO

Integrating Vegetables And Fruits

A fundamental component of a diet that combats inflammation is the liberal consumption of fruits and vegetables. Consuming these nutrient-dense foods provides individuals with rheumatoid arthritis with an abundance of health benefits, including inflammation management and overall health enhancement.

1. An abundance of antioxidants: Vegetables and fruits are a rich source of antioxidants, which assist the body in neutralizing free

radicals. The generation of free radicals during inflammation has the potential to cause cellular damage and exacerbate the progression of rheumatoid arthritis. A dietary regimen that includes an assortment of vibrant fruits and vegetables may help individuals with rheumatoid arthritis fortify their antioxidant defenses.

2. Rich in Fiber Composition: A wide variety of fruits and vegetables are dietary fiber powerhouses. In addition to promoting digestive health, fiber possesses anti-inflammatory properties. It contributes to the

regulation of blood sugar levels, which is an essential factor in weight management for individuals with rheumatoid arthritis (RA), given that obesity can worsen joint discomfort.

3. Omega-3 oily Acids: Although predominantly present in oily fish, omega-3 fatty acids are also present in flaxseeds and hazelnuts, among other fruits and vegetables. It has been demonstrated that these essential lipids possess anti-inflammatory properties, which may reduce joint inflammation and alleviate the symptoms of rheumatoid arthritis.

4. Phytonutrients: An ample supply of phytonutrients—bioactive compounds associated with potential anti-inflammatory properties—can be found in fruits and vegetables. In addition to aiding in the fight against inflammation, these compounds also promote immune system health as a whole.

5. Alkalising Impact: Certain vegetables and fruits have an alkalising influence on the body. Although the scientific validity of the alkaline diet remains debatable, advocates propose that it might aid in inflammation reduction by establishing an

environment that is less favorable to inflammatory mechanisms.

In summary, the control of Rheumatoid Arthritis necessitates more than just pharmacological approaches; an anti-inflammatory dietary regimen, notably one abundant in fruits and vegetables, possesses tremendous potential for promoting a favorable progression of the condition. By developing an awareness of the correlation between dietary selections, RA, inflammation, and the former, individuals can make educated decisions that promote their well-being and health as a whole.

In addition to adding diversity and flavor to daily meals, the inclusion of fruits and vegetables provides a natural and delectable method to combat the underlying inflammatory processes associated with RA. With the continuous advancement of research in this domain, the incorporation of an anti-inflammatory diet into a holistic strategy for managing Rheumatoid Arthritis may grow in significance, enabling individuals to assume a proactive stance regarding their well-being and standard of living.

In contemporary society, where refined foods and sedentary

lifestyles predominate, it is impossible to exaggerate the significance of maintaining joint health. Proper maintenance is necessary for the optimal functioning of our joints, which are complex intersections of bones that grant us mobility. In addition to traditional medical interventions, the foods we ingest also constitute a substantial component of joint health. By incorporating a diet abundant in lean proteins, whole cereals, and healthy lipids, we can significantly enhance the health of our joints and foster general wellness.

An Overview of Lean Proteins: Proteins serve as fundamental components of life, and integrating lean sources into one's protein intake can offer notable advantages for joint health. Lean protein sources, including poultry, fish, legumes, and tofu, offer vital amino acids while excluding the surplus saturated lipids that are present in certain types of red meats.

A Grilled Lemon Herb Chicken recipe presents a palatable method of incorporating lean protein into one's dietary regimen. This culinary creation, when marinated in a mixture of citrus, garlic, and herbs, not only satisfies the senses but also imparts beneficial anti-inflammatory properties to the joints.

Due to its high protein content and minimal calorie content, chicken breast is an excellent option for individuals seeking joint support.

Quinoa and Black Bean Salad: Consider a Quinoa and Black Bean Salad as a plant-based protein option. Black beans and quinoa, both of which are complete proteins, are combined to produce a dish rich in nutrients, including magnesium, a mineral recognized for its possible anti-inflammatory properties. The incorporation of fresh vegetables contributes a vibrant hue and supplementary vitamins that are beneficial for the joints.

Salmon with Dill in the oven: Salmon, being abundant in omega-3 fatty acids, is an exceptional option for enhancing joint health.

A recipe for Baked Salmon with Dill not only produces a delectable and savory dish but also incorporates vital omega-3 fatty acids, which have been associated with a decrease in bodily inflammation. The recipe's simplicity serves to emphasize that fortifying joints can be prepared in a straightforward and delectable manner.

CHAPTER THREE

Whole Grains For Meals Rich In Nutrients

Comprehending the Function of Whole Grains: An essential component of a diet that is kind to joints, whole cereals provide an array of nutrients including fiber, vitamins, and minerals. In contrast to refined grains, whole grains maintain their bran and germ layers, thereby offering a heightened nutritional composition that potentially promotes joint health.

Stir-Fried Vegetables with Brown Rice: A vibrant and nourishing method of integrating whole grains into a dish is by preparing a vegetable stir-fry with brown rice. Brown rice, classified as a whole grain, is an excellent source of fiber and manganese, an essential mineral for joint health that is believed to promote cartilage formation. When accompanied by a variety of fresh vegetables, this dish possesses not only aesthetic appeal but also a wealth of nutrients that are beneficial for the joints.

The recipe for Quinoa Stuffed Bell Peppers features quinoa earning a second appearance. By combining this adaptable whole grain with lean minced turkey, a filling is produced that is abundant in essential amino acids and protein. Bell peppers improve joint health through the consumption of vitamin C, which is recognized for its potential involvement in the synthesis of collagen, an essential constituent of joint tissues.

Oatmeal with Berries and Nuts: Begin the day with a warm bowl of oatmeal garnished with berries and nuts for a joint-healthy start. Whole grains, including oats, are an excellent source of beta-glucans, a fiber variety that may possess anti-inflammatory properties. Berries, which are abundant in beneficial lipids, and almonds, which are loaded with antioxidants, harmonize in flavor to promote joint health.

Healthy Fats And Dishes Rich In Omega-3

The Critical Role of Nutritious Fats: In contrast to the fallacious belief that all lipids are harmful, healthful fats are indispensable for the maintenance of overall health, which includes proper joint function. The integration of monounsaturated and polyunsaturated fat sources into one's diet, including avocados, olive oil, and rich salmon, may yield beneficial outcomes concerning joint health.

Avocado and Chickpea Salad: In addition to introducing healthy lipids, a variety of nutrients that are beneficial to joint health are included in a refreshing avocado and chickpea salad. Avocados contain an abundance of monounsaturated lipids, whereas chickpeas provide protein and fiber derived from plants. By combining these components, a gratifying salad is produced that promotes joint health and general wellness.

Skewers of Mediterranean Grilled Vegetables Drizzled in Olive Oil: A gustatory experience reminiscent of the Mediterranean is facilitated by olive oil-drizzled grilled vegetable skewers. An essential component of the Mediterranean diet, olive oil is rich in monounsaturated lipids and has been linked to potential anti-inflammatory effects. Served alongside an assortment of grilled vegetables in a rainbow hue, this dish not only provides a gustatory delight but also epitomizes the benefits of nourishing joints.

Try Walnut-Crusted Baked Cod, a delectable dish that is abundant in omega-3 fatty acids. An essential omega-3 fatty acid known as alpha-linolenic acid (ALA), which is found in walnuts, is utilized to season a baked cod crust with flavor. The omega-3 fatty acids found in cod and walnuts may aid in the reduction of inflammation, which is advantageous for joint health.

Adopting a dietary regimen that primarily consists of lean proteins, whole cereals, and healthy lipids is both palatable and functional in its objective of promoting joint health. These recipes demonstrate a commitment to both gastronomic satisfaction and joint health. It is essential to seek personalized advice from a healthcare professional before making any culinary choices that may contribute to a healthy lifestyle. This consultation is particularly valuable in addressing specific health concerns and requirements. Choosing palatable and healthful foods that nourish the joints is a stride toward a more active and vibrant lifestyle.

Managing rheumatoid arthritis (RA) effectively frequently necessitates adjustments to one's lifestyle and diet, in addition to the use of medications, due to the unique difficulties associated with this condition. A crucial component of this comprehensive methodology entails the integration of anti-inflammatory components into one's daily dietary regimen. This exhaustive manual will delve into fundamental principles including refreshment suggestions, deserts incorporating anti-inflammatory components, and pragmatic meal planning advice specifically designed to assist individuals in managing the intricacies of rheumatoid arthritis.

CHAPTER FOUR

Joint Health-Promoting

Anti-Inflammatory

Beverages

Frequently, the pursuit of joint health commences with dietary choices. Anti-inflammatory beverages are of paramount importance in facilitating the management of rheumatoid arthritis by offering relief and support. Green tea, which is abundant in polyphenols and possesses powerful anti-inflammatory attributes, emerges as a preferred option. It has been demonstrated that these polyphenols, specifically epigallocatechin gallate (EGCG), can regulate immune responses, which may result in a reduction of joint inflammation.

Golden milk and other beverages infused with turmeric are also delicious additions to an arthritis-friendly regimen. Curcumin, the bioactive constituent present in turmeric, demonstrates potent antioxidant and anti-inflammatory properties, thereby providing organic alleviation for inflammation and joint discomfort.

In addition, the inclusion of raw ginger or ginger tea in one's regimen confers an extra anti-inflammatory enhancement. Ginger, which is rich in the analgesic and anti-inflammatory compound gingerol, is an excellent addition to the diet of individuals in search of all-natural remedies for joint pain.

Maintaining Body Nutrition Between Meals

The selection of munchies is of paramount importance in sustaining energy levels over the day, and individuals diagnosed with rheumatoid arthritis can improve their overall joint health by judiciously selecting refreshments. It is crucial to choose foods that are rich in nutrients and have anti-inflammatory properties.

It is advisable to include walnuts or almonds in your regular refreshment rotation. Omega-3 fatty acids, which are abundant in these almonds, have been associated with decreased inflammation and enhanced joint health. Moreover, these almonds offer a gratifying texture and can be effortlessly combined with freshly harvested fruit to create a pleasurable and nourishing nibble.

Berry fruits, including blueberries and strawberries, are rich in anti-inflammatory antioxidants and are also quite tasty. Consider combining them with yogurt to create a satiating and joint health-promoting snack that is anti-inflammatory and refreshing.

Another nutrient-dense and versatile option is avocado, which can be pureed and spread on whole-grain crackers. Lower levels of inflammatory markers have been linked to the monounsaturated fats found in avocados; therefore, these lipids are an excellent option for those who are managing rheumatoid arthritis.

Desserts Containing Anti-Inflammatory Components

Dessert consumption is not necessarily forbidden for individuals with rheumatoid arthritis. Desserts that contain anti-inflammatory components have the potential to be both delectable and beneficial for joint health.

Dark chocolate, due to its substantial cocoa content,

comprises flavonoids which are known to exhibit antioxidant and anti-inflammatory characteristics. Snacking on a modest portion of dark chocolate can provide an indulgence that is guilt-free and beneficial to one's overall health.

Almond milk-based chia seed pudding adorned with fresh berries is an additional delectable dessert alternative. Omega-3 fatty acids and fiber are abundant in chia seeds, which not only provide a gratifying snack but also promote joint health.

By integrating turmeric into confection recipes, one can

imaginatively capitalize on the anti-inflammatory properties it possesses. For a culinary experience that is also beneficial for the joints, contemplate incorporating turmeric into your preferred dessert recipes creating cookies infused with turmeric, or adding a pinch of turmeric to your desserts.

CHAPTER FIVE

Meal Planning Suggestions for a Diet-Friendly to Rheumatoid Arthritis

Developing a meal plan that places joint health as a priority necessitates careful deliberation regarding meal composition and constituents. The following are pragmatic meal preparation suggestions customized to promote a diet tolerant to rheumatoid arthritis:

1. Adopt an Omega-3 Fatty Acid Diet: Incorporate omega-3 fatty acid sources into your diet, such as

flaxseeds, chia seeds, and fatty fish (salmon, mackerel, sardines), to aid in the reduction of joint inflammation.

2. Plate Decade: To guarantee a varied assortment of antioxidants and anti-inflammatory compounds, select an assortment of vibrant fruits and vegetables. A more vibrant plate corresponds to a more favorable nutritional profile.

3. Whole Grains: Opt for whole grains as opposed to refined grains, such as brown rice, quinoa, and oatmeal. Whole cereals furnish vital nutrients and dietary

fiber, thereby potentially mitigating inflammation and promoting digestive health.

4. Protein Intake: Give precedence to lean protein sources, including poultry, tofu, and legumes, to promote muscle health while minimizing pro-inflammatory effects.

5. Conscientious Cooking Techniques: Select cooking approaches that maintain the nutritional value of the components. Grilling, roasting, and steaming are all superior alternatives to frying.

6. It is vital to maintain proper hydration to safeguard joint health. Herbal infusions and water have the potential to enhance general health and facilitate the body's innate physiological functions.

Concluding Remarks: Facilitating Your Pathway to Joint Health

A mindful meal plan and the consumption of anti-inflammatory beverages, munchies, and desserts can contribute substantially to the management of rheumatoid arthritis. By exercising self-control over the foods you ingest, you enable yourself to provide nourishment for your joints as well as your body.

It is imperative to seek guidance from healthcare professionals or nutritionists to customize dietary decisions to suit specific requirements and guarantee their congruence with the overarching treatment strategy. By adopting a holistic perspective on nutrition, one can initiate a process of bolstering joint health by indulging in the benefits of anti-inflammatory components and advancing general wellness.

www.ingramcontent.com/pod-product-compliance
Lightning Source LLC
Chambersburg PA
CBHW071040260726
48661CB00007B/3075